AF483772

Hardcover ISBN: 979-8-218-16891-9

First hardcopy edition April 2023.

Super Creative
www.supercreative.global

In everybody's consciousness, the **last** thing usually comes to mind **first**. A film is the result of years of hard work by hundreds of people, but we only think of the 2 hours on screen. A special event seems to be just one night only, but is born from months of planning, budgeting, calls, vendors, wrong specifications and adjusting on the fly. This journey that you are embarking on will be no different.

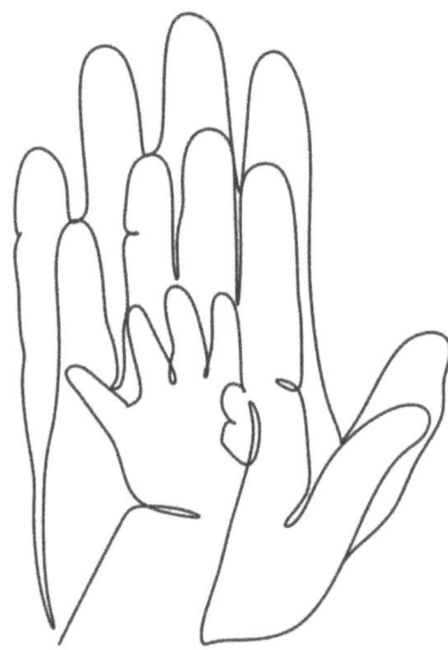

That's why I started this journal with the last thing: a blank space for **your baby's name**. It will seem like an impossible task at times and I'm not going to lie, for some it will be. My hope is that with the help of this journal, you will one day be able to complete the first and most important thing in this book: the cover.

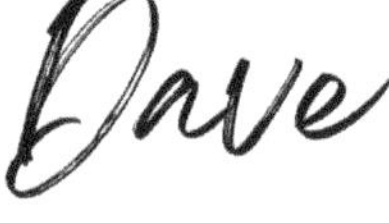

PERSONAL INFORMATION

In case of loss, please return to one of us below.

Intended Parent #1	Intended Parent #2
Name	Name
Phone	Phone
Email	Email
Address	Address

Family Doctor

Phone

Address

Our 'Why'

MY WHY

I wrote this journal because I realized that there were plenty of pregnancy and surrogacy journals that were aimed at straight couples, but there were no resources for gay men. We've been excluded enough, so I'm changing that today.

The aim of this journal is to guide you through the most incredible project you will undertake in your life: creating a baby through surrogacy. I'm not going to lie to you... It will be full of trepidation, worry, tears and hardship. But, it will also be full of hope, wonder, thankfulness and joy.

By writing this, I hope to show you that **two gay men having a baby through surrogacy is possible**.

HOW TO USE THIS BOOK

The hardest and most rewarding journey is ahead of you. And, you have taken the first step. Congratulations!

I know that everyone learns, works and plans differently, so there are a range of page formats for you to use: lined, grids, prompted questionnaires, pictures, even spaces to cut and fold. Use what works for you!

I've combined the **practical** with the **emotional** concerns that have come up in our own journey to fatherhood. We have grown so much as people and feel that fully engaging with both aspects of this journey made us stronger and a better team.

To that end, I have broken the process down into stages and given you **prompts** and **questions** to think about throughout each phase.

Everybody's journey is personal and different. If your path takes you out of order or you don't have some of the steps or you undertake extra steps, don't feel like this is unusual. Depending on whether your journey is in your home country or a foreign one, with a known Egg Donor or through an agency, with an incredible friend or relative as your Gestational Carrier or with a new friend, you will have more or fewer decisions to make.

I have aimed to capture as much as is common, but if your journey takes you outside these bounds, I have **blank pages** in each chapter for you to use. Just know that it makes your journey all the more special.

Because I love a good celebration, I've included **milestone achievements** throughout the journey with space to document that win. Be sure to celebrate individual moments - you've earned it!

I hope this journal becomes your guide and can one day turn into a keepsake for your precious little one when they are emotionally ready.

Big hugs and love - good luck on your journey.

IMPORTANT NOTES

- Nothing in this journal constitutes legal advice, therapy or instruction in any form. The purpose of this publication is merely to prompt you to do your own thinking.

- I have used the gender neutral pronouns **they/them** when referring to Egg Donors and Gestational Carriers. This decision was made as I want to remain inclusive to all people who may be involved in this wondrous journey.
- This journal follows the path of a Gestational Carrier surrogacy journey. That is, your Egg Donor and your Gestational Carrier are different people. People using other methods of surrogacy may still find this journal helpful, however, some elements will be applicable to you while others may be missing.
- Lastly, this journal is written to help gay couples work through the process of a GC surrogacy journey. It's pretty specific, honestly, and that was purposeful, because there are a lot of distinct steps that only need to be taken by gay couples throughout this process. That being said, my intention is not to add to the exclusionary history of other marginalized groups. So, I have a plan!

WHAT'S NEXT?

My hope is that with the proceeds of this journal, I can expand upon a range of items that can include other marginalized groups that want to have babies. Through consultation with lesbian couples, single men and women, trans people and more, I want to be able to authentically help in the same way that I am with gay couples.

From there, inclusive children's books, apparel, who knows!

You can support or follow my journey on my website, Amazon Author page or on all of the socials. Check them all out here:

CONTENTS

1 Research

21 Budget

35 Embryo Creation

65 Surrogacy

117 Birthday Party

129 Notes

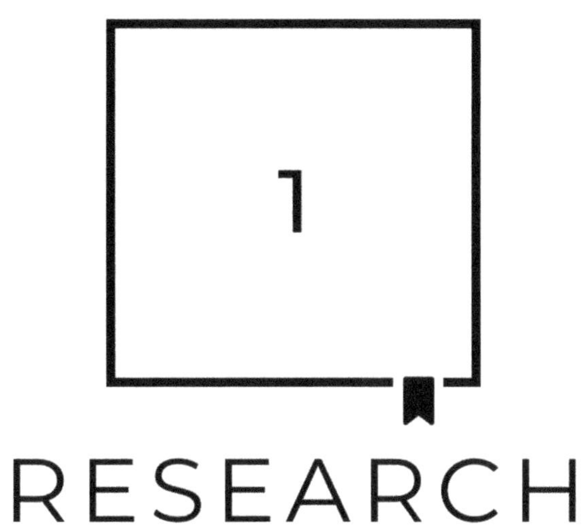

RESEARCH

Let's start at the very beginning...

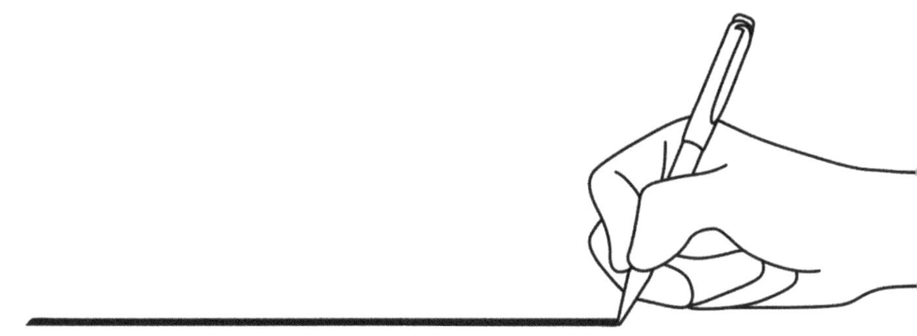

A very good place to start is to figure out what options are available to you. Once you start looking in to it, things can quickly feel overwhelming. It's almost like there are infinite possibilities, but yet there are so few solid answers.

Because there are so many options, my advice is to delve deep, as the right option for you might only come up with a little digging. On the following pages, I've given you some prompts to help you ask yourselves the right questions. From there, you can start asking others the right questions.

Just remember this: there is no single answer for everyone.

BASIC DEFINITIONS

Intended Parent (IP)	You two! The people who become the legal parent of a child born through surrogacy.
Egg Donor (ED)	A person who donates eggs to enable another person to have a child.
Gestational Carrier (GC)	A person who carries and delivers a child for somebody else. The current term for a surrogate.
Known	An Egg Donor who you already have a relationship with (relative, friend, etc.)
Anonymous	An Egg Donor selected through an agency without identifying information.
Independent	An Egg Donor or Gestational Carrier who you seek out without the help of an agency.

THE BASICS

Let's begin with logistics. Each of you should consider these questions and fill them out independently. Your definitions of the below terms may differ, as industry standards differ also. Start with IP#2 then fold the page along the line above, so the answers remain hidden. Once you're both done, regroup and discuss.

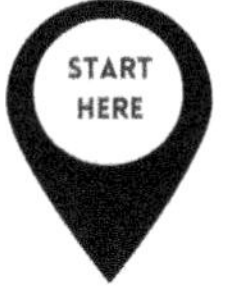

	Intended Parent #1	Intended Parent #2
Name		
How many kids total?		
How many kids this journey?		
If more than one, through twin journey or multiple GCs?		
Gender Preference?		

Egg Donor:

Agency vs. Independent		
Known vs. Anonymous		

Gestational Carrier:

Agency vs. Independent		

Sperm Contributor:

Who? Both?		

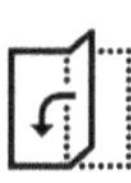

CONFERENCES & EDUCATION

There are many conferences and virtual education options out there that tackle surrogacy, sometimes specifically for gay men. Make a list below and try to attend at least one. That education will prove invaluable.

CONFERENCE NOTES

Conference Name: Date:

Useful Takeaways:

Contacts Made:

(add to Important Contacts in Chapter 6)

CONFERENCE NOTES

Conference Name: Date:

Useful Takeaways:

Contacts Made:

(add to Important Contacts in Chapter 6)

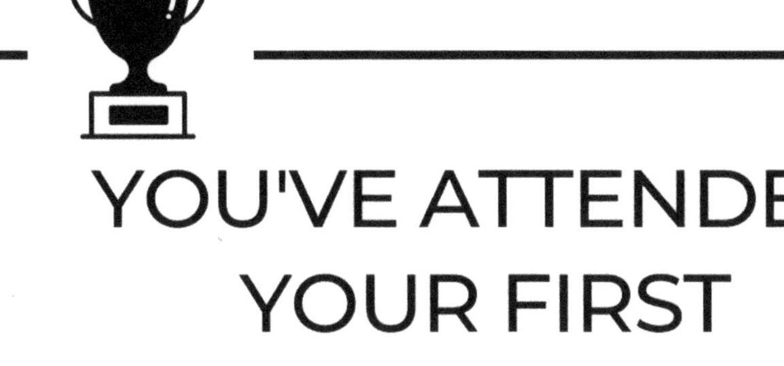

YOU'VE ATTENDED YOUR FIRST CONFERENCE

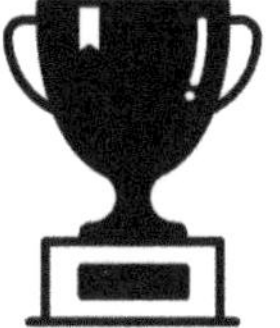

CONGRATULATIONS!

Date

That's a big (sometimes overwhelming) first step in
educating yourself.

SUPPORT GROUPS

Online and in-person support groups exist through social media and in communities around the globe. Do some research to find groups that you can join and build a network of support.

COUNTRIES

Different countries have different laws about same sex surrogacy. While there are ways to go through the process in many countries, be sure that you fully understand the immigration, legal, ethical, travel, medical and insurance implications of your decision, as well as many other factors such a political stability. Use the space below to list out pros and cons of each.

QUESTIONS GALORE

As you start your planning, it's important to consider logistical, ethical and financial aspects and be sure you're both in lock step. Some prompts are below:

Personal and Ethical

What would you like your relationship to be like with your ED and GC? Consider pre-, during and post-procedure.

How do you feel about the ethics of the surrogacy process within the country that you are considering?

Is the GC adequately compensated and protected from exploitation?

How can you ensure that the GC is fully informed and consenting?

Are there any peculiarities in this locale that require added discretion? How do you feel about this?

What is the story that you want to tell your child when they can understand?

Clinics

What is your process and what are the steps?

What is your success rate?

What are the costs associated with procedures and what happens if there are complications?

What are the risks associated with the procedures?

Can you provide references?

What are your communication protocols and what support will we receive?

Does the country or state that you are located in have particular laws or requirements?

Agencies

What is your process and what are the steps?

What is your average waiting time for a match?

What happens in the case of a failed surrogacy attempt?

What psychological evaluations and support do you provide?

CLINICS

Clinics are the medical providers who perform the procedures necessary for your particular journey. Many things happen there such as testing of the sperm contributor and ED, ultrasounds, egg retrieval and embryo transfer. There are clinics all over the world, however, keep in mind that different countries and even states have their own rules around same sex surrogacy. In some countries, clinics and agencies are housed under the same roof which brings some additional pros and cons to consider. Research who's who and list your findings below.

AGENCIES

Egg Donor Agencies connect (a.k.a. match) Intended Parents (IPs) with Egg Donors (EDs). Surrogacy agencies match IPs with Gestational Carriers (GCs). You can choose to use agencies or source an ED or GC yourself through your personal relationships or online. Regardless of your choice, ensure that you educate yourselves about the legal, ethical, medical and psychological implications of the surrogacy relationship. ED and GC matching can sometimes be provided by the same agency and even your clinic may have available donors. Use the below to explore who's out there.

LEGAL BASICS

Here are some questions to consider as you build out your plan. Your legal team will be able to advise you further on these questions, but use them to start thinking about the larger issues before you get into the nitty gritty.

Jurisdiction

In which country and city are we planning on undertaking each stage of this journey? Consider where you live, where the ED lives, where the clinic is, where the surrogate lives, where they will give birth. Sometimes where the embryo transfer takes place can give flexibility and other times not, for example.

What are the laws and regulations around this journey in this jurisdiction?

If both of you cannot be listed, who will be on the birth certificate?

Do I require a Pre-Birth or Post-Birth Order?

Will I require immigration assistance?

Relationship and Responsibility

Will either your ED or GC be known to you?

Are there any fees that will be paid to either your ED or GC or is this altruistic?

What are our responsibilities as IPs?

What are the responsibilities of your ED and GC?

If you are unable to reach the hospital in time for the birth, what should happen?

Health and Future

What insurance needs to be obtained and what might existing insurance cover?

How do you feel about terminating pregnancies when medically necessary?

What will happen if one or both of you pass away?

What will happen if you break up?

What should happen to any remaining embryos after this journey?

How are your parental rights protected?

RESOURCES

Here's a list of fantastic websites for you to begin your research. Read as much as you can and add in any resources you may come across below.

Men Having Babies	https://menhavingbabies.org/
Gays with Kids	https://gayswithkids.com/
Surrogacy Dictionary	https://www.gostork.com/blog/surrogacy/surrogacy-guide-all-the-terms/
We are Donor Conceived	https://www.wearedonorconceived.com/
We are Egg Donors	https://www.weareeggdonors.com/
Gay Parents To Be	https://www.gayparentstobe.com/

<table><tr><td>JAN</td><td>FEB</td><td>MAR</td><td>APR</td><td>MAY</td><td>JUN</td><td>JUL</td><td>AUG</td><td>SEP</td><td>OCT</td><td>NOV</td><td>DEC</td></tr></table>

1 2 3 4 5 6 7 8 9 10 11 12 13 14 15 16 17 18 19 20 21 22 23 24 25 26 27 28 29 30 31

Free journaling pages

JAN	FEB	MAR	APR	MAY	JUN	JUL	AUG	SEP	OCT	NOV	DEC

1 2 3 4 5 6 7 8 9 10 11 12 13 14 15 16 17 18 19 20 21 22 23 24 25 26 27 28 29 30 31

RESEARCH

JAN	FEB	MAR	APR	MAY	JUN	JUL	AUG	SEP	OCT	NOV	DEC

1 2 3 4 5 6 7 8 9 10 11 12 13 14 15 16 17 18 19 20 21 22 23 24 25 26 27 28 29 30 31

MENTAL HEALTH CHECK IN

Date

Top 3 things we achieved:

Most rewarding thing:

We have felt:

Our three most dominant emotions were:

We are grateful for:

We rate this time period as:

We are working on:

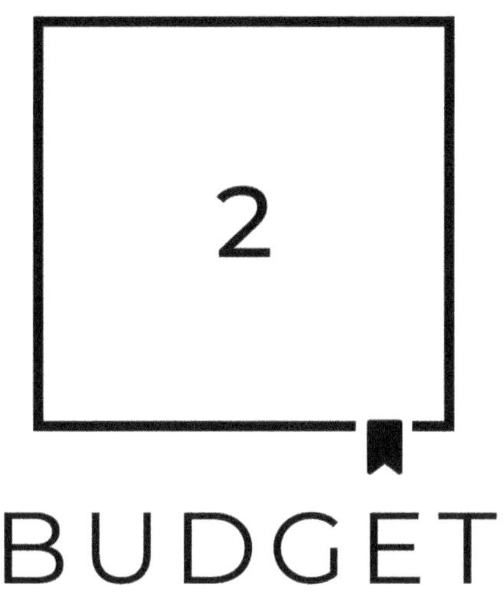

BUDGET

Dollar dollar bills... Keep them in check!

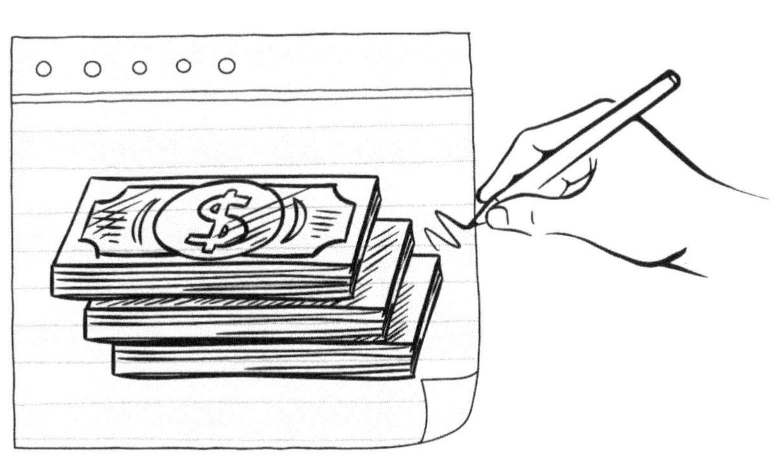

This is where things get real. When you're trying to understand how much this whole process could cost, keep in mind that there are many ways that surrogacy can be achieved but also know that you are dealing with biology. Things will almost certainly change and shift as you progress through the process and, as such, so will your timelines and budget.

Your research in the previous chapter will help you build your budget, however, always build contingencies in to your plan.

One piece of advice that made sense to us was to think about the whole journey as an amalgamation of a few stages. You can complete a stage at a time and then stop and regroup to make the entirety more manageable.

BASIC CHRONOLOGY

Screening	Checking yourselves out to clear you medically and psychologically for this journey.
Legal	Recruiting solid representation so that you are clear and comfortable about your and other parties' responsibilities.
Embryo Creation	The process of fertilizing donor eggs with one or both IPs sperm in order to create and store your embryos. Includes medical, genetic and psychological screening and legal for your egg donor, as applicable.
Surrogacy	The process of transfering your embryo/s into your Gestational Carrier (GC) and the ensuing pregnancy. Includes screening and legal for your GC, as well as any concerns about bringing your baby home, as applicable.

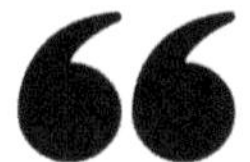

"THOSE WHO SAY IT CAN'T BE DONE ARE USUALLY INTERRUPTED BY OTHERS DOING IT."

Found in a fortune cookie, 2009

This single quote has pushed us to do "impossible" things throughout our entire lives. From moving countries to starting new careers to pursuing surrogacy, these words helped us persevere.

We hope they do the same for you.

Big love and hugs,
Dave + Mathew

BUDGET BASICS

Here are some questions to consider as you build your budget.

How will you fund this? Savings, a loan, family support?

In which country would you like to undertake surrogacy?

Are you compensating an ED or GC?

Are you using an agency for either of the above?

How many embryos would you transfer at once? Consider the higher risks associated with multiple embryo transfers.

Is your ideal clinic nearby or do you need to have a travel line item?

Do you, your ED or GC have insurance that might help?

Do you have enough contingency funds in case something goes wrong?

Some points that you should be aware of:

- Most clinics and surrogacy agencies will provide you with estimated fees and expenses. Be sure to compare.
- While budget is hugely important, it's also vital to consider the reputation of the team that you are building including the clinic, agencies, legal, etc.
- Your clinic will be part of both the egg donation and surrogacy stages and you will have costs for both stages to account for.
- There are organizations in many countries that provide grants, discounts and funding as well as employers who have fertility programs that might help.
- Each party in this process should have their own legal representation, psychological and medical assessments. You will be responsible for all fees.
- Medications and additional testing of embryos are not insubstantial costs. Be sure to research these.
- If anything were to go wrong with any of the procedures, you are generally responsible to help monetarily.
- GCs are generally compensated a fee and also require to be supported with payments for lost wages, maternity clothing and travel, for example.
- You will generally need to open an escrow account for payments to your ED and GC which will demand some fees. Your legal team can help set this up, or you can research your own trust company.

GRANTS AND FUNDING

Research different ways to help you fund your journey. Some not-for-profit organizations offer grants and discounts, financial institutions sometimes offer IVF or fertility loans, even your clinic might have options to help tackle the financial mountain.

BUDGET BUILDING BLOCKS

To help you break this down, I have listed the major stages of the process below along with starter items. Feel free to take notes against any of those stages and build out additional line items as the basis for your budget.

Screening	Psychological Screenings (IPs/ED/GC)	
	Genetic Screening (IP/ED)	
	Medical Screening (IP/ED/GC)	
Legal	Legal Representation (IPs/ED/GC)	
	Court Filings/Immigration	
General	Trust/Escrow Account	
Embryo Creation	Clinic Fees and Procedures	
	Agency Fees	
	Medications	
	Insurance	
	Travel (ED/IPs)	
	Embryo Testing	
	Contingency for Complications	
Surrogacy	Agency Fees	
	GC Compensation	
	GC Expenses and Lost Wages	
	Medications	
	Insurance	
	Travel (GC, partner (if applicable), IPs)	
	Hospital Fees	
	Contingency for Complications	

BUDGET

Build your budget on the following pages. Remember that this is a starting point and it will continue to evolve. Clinics and agencies will provide estimates that can help you here.

Item	Notes	Price	Qty	Total

BUDGET CONT.

Item	Notes	Price	Qty	Total

BUDGET CONT.

Item	Notes	Price	Qty	Total

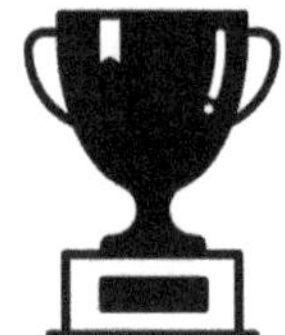

YOU'VE COMPLETED YOUR BUDGET

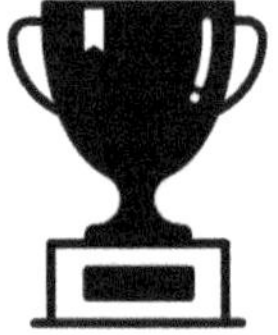

CONGRATULATIONS!

Date

That can be a big, scary number. Break it down into stages, if you can. But, also note that the budget will continue to evolve and shift as biology does its thing.

You've got this!

| JAN | FEB | MAR | APR | MAY | JUN | JUL | AUG | SEP | OCT | NOV | DEC |

1 2 3 4 5 6 7 8 9 10 11 12 13 14 15 16 17 18 19 20 21 22 23 24 25 26 27 28 29 30 31

BUDGET

MENTAL HEALTH CHECK IN

Date _______________________

Top 3 things we achieved:

____

____

____

We have felt:

Most rewarding thing:

Our three most dominant emotions were:

We are grateful for:

We rate this time period as:

We are working on:

____

____

____

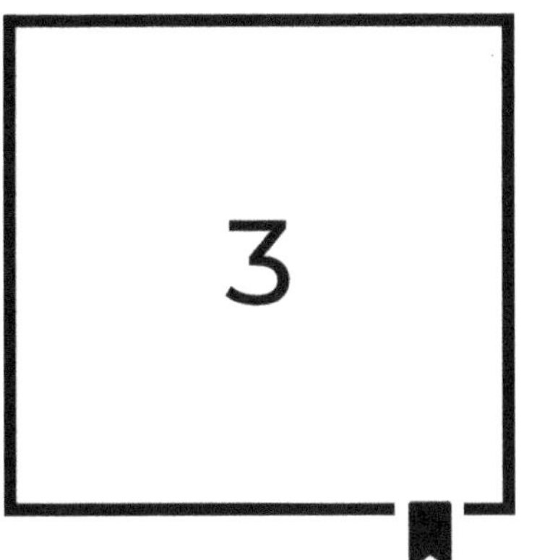

EMBRYO CREATION

It takes a team. Let's build one.

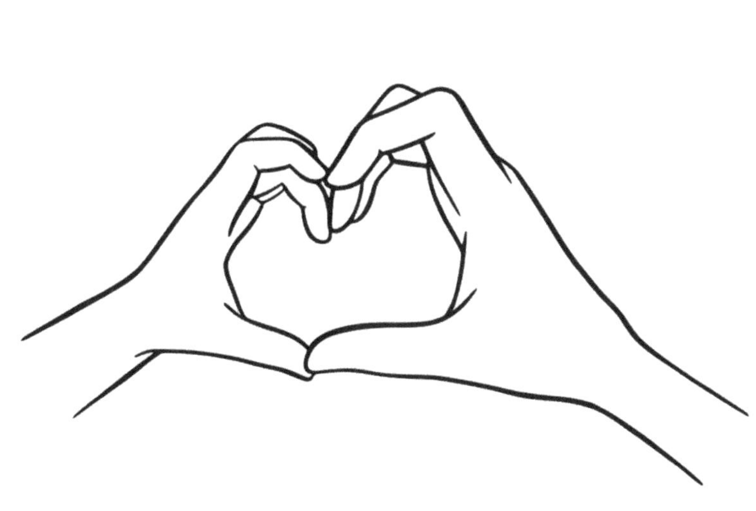

This stage of the process comes with a lot of decisions and selections as you build the team that will support you throughout your journey. It contains a lot of screenings, legalese and paperwork along with more information that will, at times, feel overwhelming.

It's also okay if it seems like one of you is impatient while the other is just struggling to keep up. Use the Mental Health Check In pages to be honest with yourselves and help you communicate your feelings with each other. This is a massive undertaking and you are brave for even getting this far.

For simplicity's sake, I have included the screening and legal processes for you and your egg donor within this Egg Donation chapter. Your clinic may have some connections to lawyers and psychologists/counselors who can perform some of these services, but do your own independent research as you build your team, too.

BASIC DEFINITIONS

Egg Retrieval	The process of removing eggs from your ED.
Assisted Reproductive Technology (ART)	A catch-all term to describe medical procedures such as IVF where eggs are fertilized by sperm in a controlled environment (test tube or petri dish).
Blastocyst	Also known as "blast" - the final stage of embryo development before transfer.
Preimplantation Genetic Testing for Aneuploidies (PGT-A)	Formerly known as Preimplantation Genetic Screening (PGS) - is used to screen embryos to ensure the correct number of chromosomes.

EMBRYO BASICS

Here are some questions to consider as you start this stage.

What is important to you when considering an egg donor? Think about genetics, health, age, personality, availability and legal considerations.

Do you know anybody who would consider being your egg donor? Would you source through an agency? Does your clinic have a database?

If considering a known donor, is this a person you want connected to your child for your entire lives?

What level of communication do you want? Pre-, during and post-retrieval?

Do you want to be updated if any new health information becomes available to them after your baby is born?

Fresh or frozen eggs? Consult your clinic for their professional advice.

Is previous experience important?

Is where they live important to you?

How is the egg donor supported through the donation process? By you, your clinic, their agency etc.

What medications need to be administered? Will you be part of that process for your known donor or will the ED take care of it?

Does your ED have a support network at home?

What does recovery look like for them? How about travel? Don't forget to include a partner, if applicable.

What extent of testing do you want the clinic to perform on the embryos?

Some points that you should be aware of:

- You can independently work with a donor, go through an agency or your clinic might have available donors. Each method has its pros and cons. I encourage you to research fully to determine which path is best for you.
- Along with selecting an egg donor, this stage includes building the first part of your team: your legal representation, psychological team, clinic and egg donor agency, as applicable.
- You will also need to pay for your ED's chosen legal representation, insurance and medical treatment, as necessary.
- Different countries (and even different states) have different laws and rules about egg donation. Be sure to research fully.

LEGAL TEAM

One of the first building blocks of your team that you should secure is your legal representation. Because of the incredibly personal nature of this process and the varying laws around the world, you will want to be as fully informed as you can. Your legal team will help with that.

As you start to research your legal team, note down what you like about them, their personality, ability to communicate on your level and your overall comfort level. Your responsibilities and all the legal documents you need to review will be much easier to digest with somebody you gel with. Some lawyers offer a flat fee for the entire process while others charge per hour worked.

Be sure to consider where you might need specialist help such as immigration, the surrogacy process, family law etc. Note that your ED and GC will require their own representation whose fees you will be responsible for. Your legal team can refer or your agencies/clinics might also have leads.

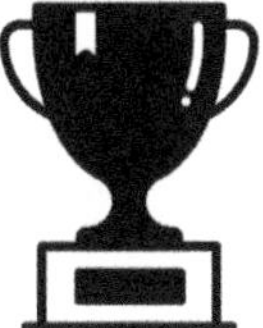

YOU'VE CONFIRMED YOUR LEGAL TEAM

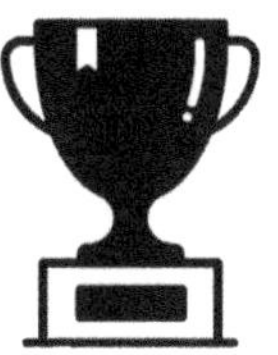

CONGRATULATIONS!

Date

You're on your way to building your complete team!

Name:

Phone:

Email:

Address:

CLINIC

List out the pros and cons of each clinic that you've shortlisted below. Note that in certain countries, agencies and clinics can be housed under one roof which can come with pros and cons.

Clinic	Pros	Cons

EGG DONOR AGENCY

List out the pros and cons of each agency that you've shortlisted below. Note that in certain countries, agencies and clinics can be housed under one roof which can come with pros and cons.

Egg Donor Agency	Pros	Cons

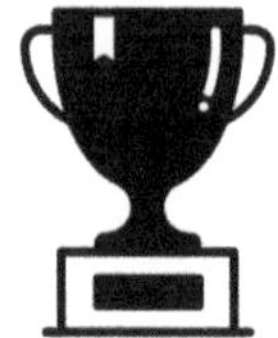

YOU'VE CONFIRMED YOUR EMBRYO TEAM

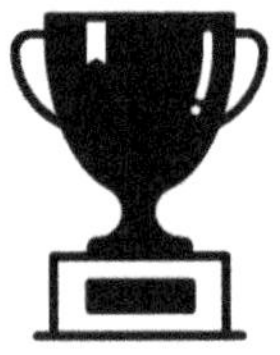

CONGRATULATIONS!

Date

You contracted your clinic and your egg donation agency
(if you needed it). Your village is growing!

SCREENINGS

Going through psychological and medical screenings can sometimes feel like you're being questioned by a detective. While it's unlikely that you 'fail' screenings (as the main purpose is to optimize the process, not disqualify), take some time to note down your experiences below and reflect.

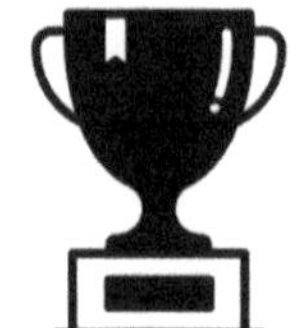

YOU'VE PASSED YOUR SCREENINGS

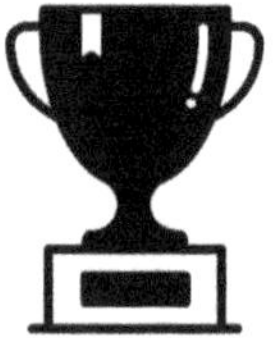

CONGRATULATIONS!

Date

Hopefully, you feel a little more ready to be dads!

TESTING
1, 2, 3

Genetic testing can be broken down into two sections: testing of the donors (both sperm and egg) and testing of the embryos themselves. In most countries, you should now have the option to test donors for genetic predisposition to a huge range of conditions. If both donors carry the recessive gene for a condition, there is a higher risk that the baby will be born with that condition. So, part of screening for ideal candidacy of egg donors is ensuring their genetics are not opening you up to additional risks.

The decision to test embryos for a multitude of genetic and other medical concerns is one that needs to be made relatively early on in the process.

Talk to your clinic about the fact that testing gives you some reassurance but will not necessarily avoid abnormalities in utero. Be sure to ask about what realistically can and cannot be determined with screening. Think about it below and, if you do decide to proceed, use the following pages to reflect on results.

Donor Testing:

TESTING 1, 2, 3 CONT.

Embryo Testing:

Decision:

TESTING 1, 2, 3 CONT.

Results:

EGG DONORS

List out your thoughts on your shortlist of egg donors below. They might be fresh or frozen donors. If you are considering a direct relationship with your egg donor (e.g. a friend or family member), pay special attention to legal, regional and ethical considerations, clear communication around financial arrangements, their home support system and their 'why' and ensure that you have medical and psychological screenings conducted. Reconsider your 'why' and the story that you'll tell your child, one day.

Egg Donor	Notes

EGG DONORS CONT.

Egg Donor	Notes

SCREENINGS

Generally, overall results of your donor's psychological and medical screenings will be shared, but the full details will not be provided to you. Sometimes, your first choice (or fifth choice) doesn't work out. Note down your feelings below.

RELATIONSHIPS

Whether your donor is known or you're just meeting them, it's important to discuss between yourselves what kind of relationship you want to have with your donor and how you will talk to family and friends about the process. Consider also what kind of relationship you want your ED to have with your child and how you will discuss the process with your child. Use the below space to reflect but also consider facilitation with a mental health professional.

Our relationship with our ED

How we will talk to family and friends about the process

RELATIONSHIPS CONT.

Our child's relationship with our ED

How we will talk to our child about the process

CONTRACTS

Should everybody be agreeable, you will begin contract negotiation which generally brings up some big (literally life or death) questions. If proceeding with a fresh cycle, at this stage, your ED will also need their own representation whose fees you are responsible for. Note down your feelings below.

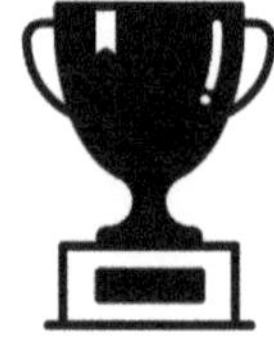

YOU'VE CONFIRMED YOUR EGG DONOR

CONGRATULATIONS!

Date

Don't count your babies before they're born, but this is a huge step!

Name:	Top 5 Reasons:
Hometown:	1.
Circle: Fresh / Frozen	2.
	3.
	4.
	5.

EGG DONATION MEDICATIONS

Medications can be scary. Especially when you read all of the potential side effects. If you are proceeding with a fresh cycle with a known donor, then as you and your ED progress and learn more, note down your feelings around the medication and procedures.

EGG DONATION CYCLE

The day has come! If you've committed to a fresh donation, your ED will visit the clinic and make sure everything is in check, then medications will begin until retrieval day. You may already have frozen sperm or you may provide your sample on the same day. While this can all feel very exciting, remember that this is biology that we're dealing with and things may not go smoothly. As you go through this process, note your emotions, tensions and reflect on your relationship below.

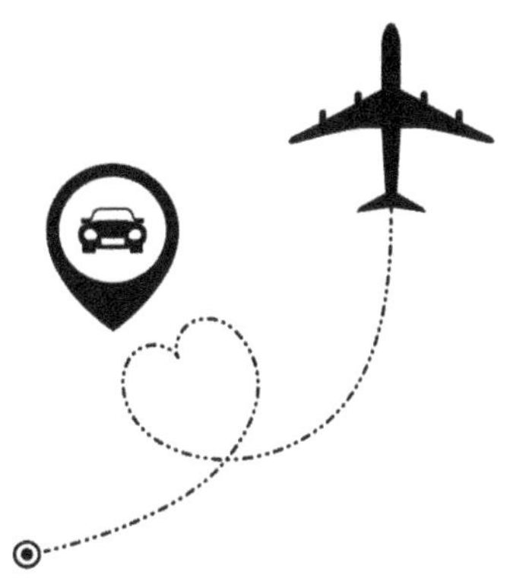

TIME TO GET ON THE ROAD!

We're headed to:

____

Because:

____

EMBRYO CREATION

Tuck your ticket stub here:

1. ✂   3. 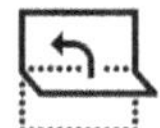   2. ✂

MORE ATTEMPTS

If things don't go exactly as intended, you may have more attempts at the embryo creation cycle. You might even have to change to a different egg donor. Use the space below to reflect.

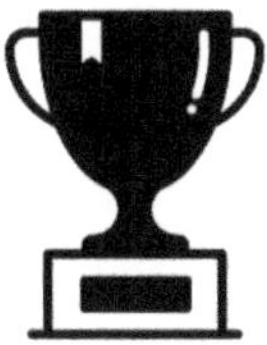

YOU'VE CREATED EMBRYOS!

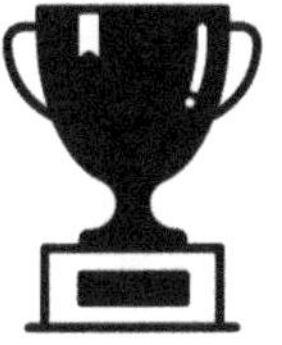

CONGRATULATIONS!

Date

This is a milestone for you! Celebrate it!

EMBRYOS!

If things have worked out, you've successfully created embryos! Take note of their details and the journey to get to them below. It may have taken multiple attempts and moments of heartbreak, but know that you've come so far. Congratulations!

No. of Eggs Retrieved	
No. of Attempts	
No. of Mature Eggs Fertilized	
No. of Embryos Frozen	
No. of Embryos Viable	
Sex (if tested)	Male: Female:
Embryo Grading	

<table><tr><td>JAN</td><td>FEB</td><td>MAR</td><td>APR</td><td>MAY</td><td>JUN</td><td>JUL</td><td>AUG</td><td>SEP</td><td>OCT</td><td>NOV</td><td>DEC</td></tr></table>

1 2 3 4 5 6 7 8 9 10 11 12 13 14 15 16 17 18 19 20 21 22 23 24 25 26 27 28 29 30 31

Genetic testing results, if applicable.

| JAN | FEB | MAR | APR | MAY | JUN | JUL | AUG | SEP | OCT | NOV | DEC |

1 2 3 4 5 6 7 8 9 10 11 12 13 14 15 16 17 18 19 20 21 22 23 24 25 26 27 28 29 30 31

MENTAL HEALTH CHECK IN

Date _______________________

Top 3 things we achieved:

____

____

____

We have felt:

Our three most dominant emotions were:

Most rewarding thing:

We are grateful for:

We rate this time period as:

We are working on:

____

____

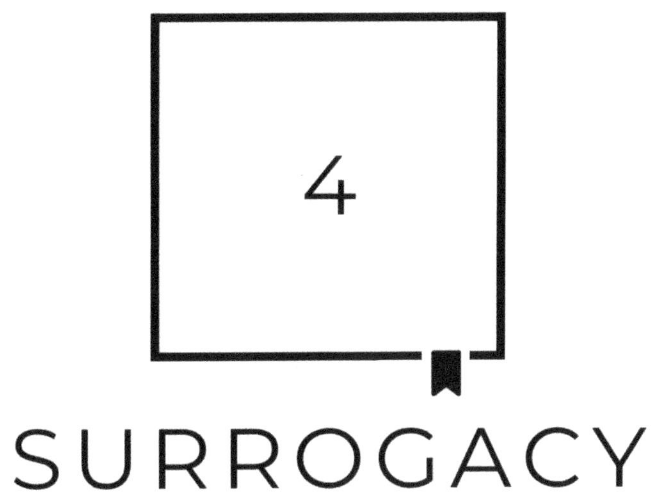

4

SURROGACY

Think sticky thoughts!

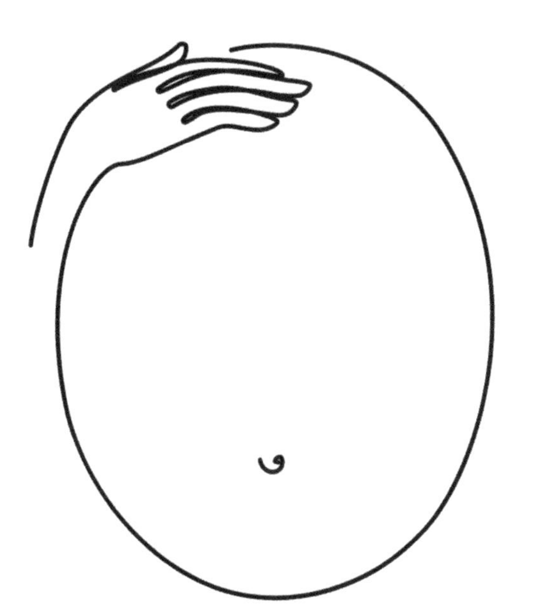

First up, let's take a second. Think about where you were a month ago, a year ago, even a couple of days ago. You might be skimming ahead and just visiting this page or you may be starting to undertake this new chapter, but reflect on just how far you've come - whether it be in knowledge, experience or even loss. Every journey has meaning and you've been creating meaning for yourselves ever since you started. Well done!

Now, onto the business end of our task at hand. It's a big one and it's okay to have some trepidation. Lean on your team for support and they will make your experience as smooth and positive as it can be. This final stage of creating your baby includes selecting the second half of your team including your GC. You'll then commence the journey to pregnancy, trimesters, hospitals and preparation for bringing your child home!

Take the time to periodically check in on each other and find new ways to support each other as your feelings develop and as you shift into prospective parents.

Big hugs and love. Good luck!

BASIC DEFINITIONS

Frozen Embryo Transfer (FET)	A fertilized and frozen embryo is thawed then transferred into your GC. This is most common, but it can be done fresh, also.
Local Monitoring Clinic	The medical facility that is close to your GC where regular appointments will occur.
Beta-hCG Testing	A blood test used to indicate pregnancy by measuring the hormone hCG. As opposed to a urine test.

SURROGACY BASICS

Here are some questions to consider as you start this stage.

What is important to you when considering a Gestational Carrier? Think about health, age, personality, availability, location, values and legal considerations.

Do you know anybody who would consider being your GC?

What kind of communication do you want with them? Will you be attending doctor's visits with them?

What is their 'why'?

What kind of relationship do you want with the GC once your child is born?

Is previous experience important?

Do you want to undertake this journey guided by an agency or independently?

Is where they live important to you?

Does your GC have a support network at home?

What does recovery look like? What about travel? Don't forget to include a partner, if applicable.

Some points that you should be aware of:

- You can independently work with a GC or go through an agency. Each method has its pros and cons. Research fully to determine which path is best for you.
- Along with selecting a GC, this stage includes building the final part of your team: your surrogacy agency, your GC's health network at home, the birth hospital.
- You will also need to pay for your GC's chosen legal representation, insurance and medical treatment, as necessary.
- Don't forget your legal team and other members of your surrogacy team are still here to support and guide you. Lean on them throughout this process for advice.
- Part way through the pregnancy, it's also time to start thinking of setting your child up for success. We have some prompts to help!
- We'll start to include more space for photos and memories as this chapter develops. This is when things start to become real!

SURROGACY AGENCY

A surrogacy agency is part of your process to help guide you, protect you and advise you on your journey with a Gestational Carrier (GC). They will help connect you with the right person to help you fulfill your dream. Just as importantly, they also protect and advise your GC.

The process looks slightly different for each agency and, depending on the state of the industry, the country and the world, wait times to match can vary greatly.

Their services go beyond matching and can include conducting medical and psychological screenings, arranging legal representation, providing financial management, coordinating appointments and offering counseling.

Note that in certain countries, agencies and clinics can be housed under one roof which can come with pros and cons.

As you start to research and interview agencies, note down your feelings and gut reactions below.

Agency	Pros	Cons

SURROGACY AGENCY CONT.

Agency	Pros	Cons

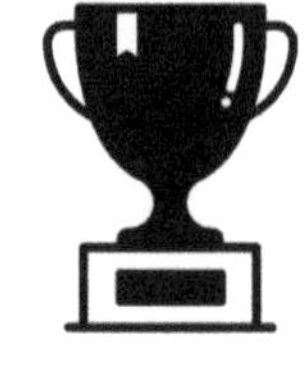

YOU'VE CONFIRMED YOUR SURROGACY AGENCY

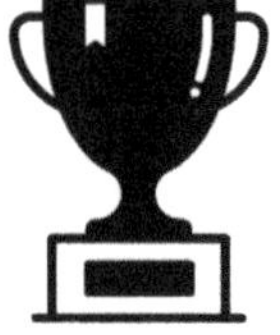

CONGRATULATIONS!

Date

Your team is building and your support network is strengthening! Go forth!

Name:

Phone:

Email:

Address:

Approximate Matching Wait:

GESTATIONAL CARRIERS

List out your thoughts on your shortlist of gestational carriers below. If you are considering an independent journey, pay special attention to legal, regional and ethical considerations, clear communication around financial arrangements, their support system and their 'why' and ensure that you have medical and psychological screenings conducted.

Gestational Carrier	Notes

GESTATIONAL CARRIERS CONT.

Gestational Carrier	Notes

RELATIONSHIPS

Whether your GC is known or you're just meeting them, it's important to discuss between yourselves what kind of relationship you want to have with them and how you will talk to family and friends about the process. Consider also what kind of relationship you want your GC to have with your child and how you will discuss the process with your child. Use the below space to reflect but also consider facilitation with a mental health professional.

Our relationship with our GC

How we will talk to family and friends about the process

RELATIONSHIPS CONT.

Our child's relationship with our GC

How we will talk to our child about the process

SCREENINGS

The results of your chosen GCs medical and psychological screenings will be shared with you. Depending on your location, more or less information will be given. Sometimes, your first choice (or fifth choice) doesn't work out. Note down your feelings below.

CONTRACTS

Should everybody be agreeable, you will begin contract negotiation which can be tumultuous or quite calm. It is normal for there to be slight tension during this period. Note down your feelings below.

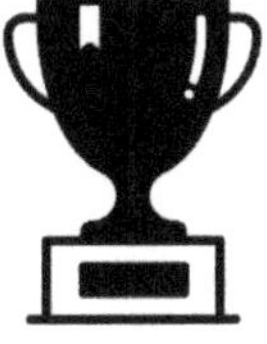

YOU'VE CONFIRMED YOUR GESTATIONAL CARRIER

CONGRATULATIONS!

Date

Oh boy, things are ramping up now!

Name:	Top 5 Reasons:
Hometown:	1.
No. of kids:	2.
	3.
	4.
	5.

SURROGACY MEDICATIONS

Medications can be scary. Especially when you read all of the potential side effects. Although it would be rare that you would be involved in the medications for your GC, note down any feelings you might have around the medication procedure.

SURROGACY

APPROACHING TRANSFER

If things have worked out, you're approaching your transfer day! There's a lot to know about how your GC is doing in the lead up to the day. Note it all down below.

Lining	
Transportation	
Medications	
Emotional Support	
Our Relationship	
Our Attendance	In Person / Video Call
Other Notes	

JAN	FEB	MAR	APR	MAY	JUN	JUL	AUG	SEP	OCT	NOV	DEC

1 2 3 4 5 6 7 8 9 10 11 12 13 14 15 16 17 18 19 20 21 22 23 24 25 26 27 28 29 30 31

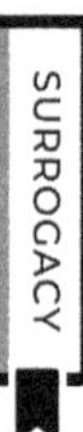

TIME TO GET ON THE ROAD!

We're headed to:

____

Because:

____

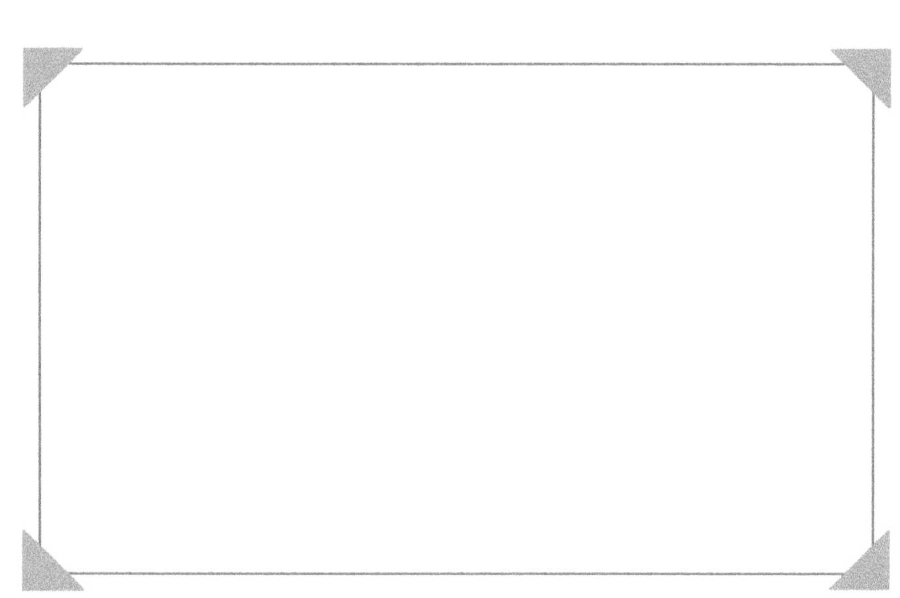

Tuck your ticket stub here:

1. ✂   3. ↰   2. ✂

MENTAL HEALTH CHECK IN

Date

Top 3 things we achieved:

Most rewarding thing:

We have felt:

Our three most dominant emotions were:

We are grateful for:

We rate this time period as:

We are working on:

TRANSFER DAY

This is monumental! Depending on your arrangement and whether you are in the same location, you may be present for the transfer day or not. Your GC will generally have some family or friends supporting them and hopefully, you can also lend your support to this exciting day.

Remember, as with the egg donation day, that this is biology that we're dealing with and things may not go smoothly.

As you go through this process, note your emotions, tensions and reflect on your relationship with each other and your GC and their loved ones below.

SURROGACY

MORE ATTEMPTS

If things don't go exactly as intended, you may have more attempts at transfer. You might even have to change to a different GC. Use the space below to reflect.

THE PREGNANCY TESTS

Aaah! Another milestone day is here.

Depending on the country and region, you may encounter blood or urine tests or both and may have follow up tests to be certain. That's generally followed by an ultrasound to confirm a heartbeat two weeks later.

Don't forget that your GC is also feeling nervous. If it helps, keep communication open and ask, for example, how they intend to remain occupied during the wait for results.

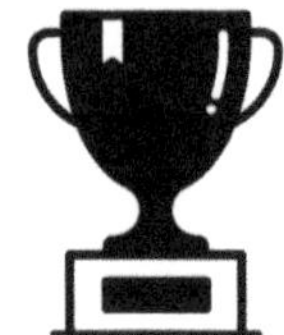

YOU'RE PREGNANT

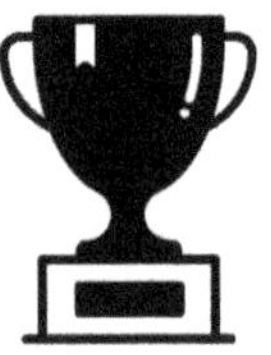

CONGRATULATIONS!

Date ___________________________

____
Due Date

A monumental moment has finally come! There's still a
journey to go, but there should definitely be hugs all
around today.

SURROGACY

THE TRIMESTERS

The fertility clinic will generally follow up with your GC until the end of the first trimester after which she will "graduate" and continue her care with her OBGYN. As your GC's pregnancy progresses, it is natural for you to feel a range of emotions and even feel conflicting thoughts, at times.
As you begin on this section of your journey, try to remain in open communication between yourselves and your GC and note how you are feeling on the following pages.
I have given you a broad range of prompts and spaces to fill along with some empty pages for you to use as you wish.

THE ULTRASOUNDS

Whether or not you are able to be at these appointments in person, your GCs medical exams, check-ins and ultrasounds are important milestones.

There are two milestone ultrasounds: the first prenatal and the anatomy ultrasound (generally done in the second trimester). There are two milestone pages dedicated to these moments coming up! Excitingly, the first ultrasound will be the first chance that you'll have to see your child! Use the following space to organize your thoughts and feelings specifically around the ultrasounds.

BABY'S FIRST ULTRASOUND

Date	
Single or multiple?	
Size	
Heartbeat	

Communication plan

What's the story we want to tell our child?

What's the story we want to tell our family and friends?

Gender Reveal?

<table>
<tr><td>JAN</td><td>FEB</td><td>MAR</td><td>APR</td><td>MAY</td><td>JUN</td><td>JUL</td><td>AUG</td><td>SEP</td><td>OCT</td><td>NOV</td><td>DEC</td></tr>
</table>

1 2 3 4 5 6 7 8 9 10 11 12 13 14 15 16 17 18 19 20 21 22 23 24 25 26 27 28 29 30 31

BABY'S SIZE CHART

Date	Weeks	Size

Our relationship with our GC...

SURROGACY

BABY'S ANATOMY ULTRASOUND

Date

Length

Weight

Notes

1 2 3 4 5 6 7 8 9 10 11 12 13 14 15 16 17 18 19 20 21 22 23 24 25 26 27 28 29 30 31

First kick! Date:

Other important milestones:

SURROGACY

SURROGACY

IT'S TIME FOR A NAME-STORM BRAINSTORM!

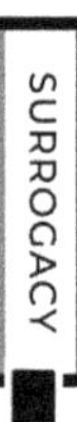

Shortlist

JAN	FEB	MAR	APR	MAY	JUN	JUL	AUG	SEP	OCT	NOV	DEC

1 2 3 4 5 6 7 8 9 10 11 12 13 14 15 16 17 18 19 20 21 22 23 24 25 26 27 28 29 30 31

Baby announcements and events

1 2 3 4 5 6 7 8 9 10 11 12 13 14 15 16 17 18 19 20 21 22 23 24 25 26 27 28 29 30 31

BABY'S ROOM & WARDROBE CHECKLIST

Tip: Shoes are just for photos until baby can walk, so don't waste too much money on them!

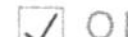 TO START   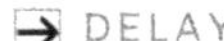 OK   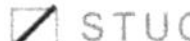 DELAY   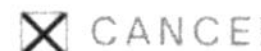 STUCK   ✕ CANCEL

JAN	FEB	MAR	APR	MAY	JUN	JUL	AUG	SEP	OCT	NOV	DEC

1 2 3 4 5 6 7 8 9 10 11 12 13 14 15 16 17 18 19 20 21 22 23 24 25 26 27 28 29 30 31

How can we support our GC during delivery?

HOSPITAL BAG CHECKLIST

Tip: Make sure you're thinking about what you'll need to bring baby home (e.g. car seat, clothes, supplies)

● TO START   ☑ OK   → DELAY   ☑ STUCK   ☒ CANCEL

TO BUY AT DESTINATION

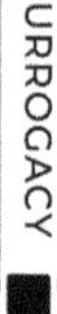

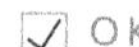 TO START 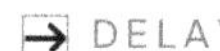 OK 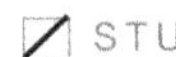 DELAY 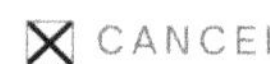 STUCK ✕ CANCEL

JAN	FEB	MAR	APR	MAY	JUN	JUL	AUG	SEP	OCT	NOV	DEC

1 2 3 4 5 6 7 8 9 10 11 12 13 14 15 16 17 18 19 20 21 22 23 24 25 26 27 28 29 30 31

Travel Plans:

(e.g. flights, accommodation, car hire)

What's in the area?

(e.g. closest groceries, restaurants, baby store, consulate)

What might be challenging in our accommodations?

(e.g. heating milk, sanitizing, laundry)

Contingencies:

(e.g. flexible fares, staying with family etc.)

<table>
<tr><td>JAN</td><td>FEB</td><td>MAR</td><td>APR</td><td>MAY</td><td>JUN</td><td>JUL</td><td>AUG</td><td>SEP</td><td>OCT</td><td>NOV</td><td>DEC</td></tr>
</table>

1 2 3 4 5 6 7 8 9 10 11 12 13 14 15 16 17 18 19 20 21 22 23 24 25 26 27 28 29 30 31

What do we need to learn?

(e.g. how to swaddle, change, bottle feed and burp)

Planning for baby to be home

Pediatricians in our area

Feeding strategy

(e.g. Breast milk delivered, formula, types and no. of bottles, sanitizers)

Safety considerations around the house

(e.g. cribs vs. baby monitors, sharp corners, trip hazards near sleeping area)

Research developmental milestones

(e.g. solid food, sleep patterns, weight)

Support groups for baby and parents

SURROGACY

What's our premature plan?

e.g. a packed hospital bag from 3rd trimester, travel and longer term accommodation, budget

HOSPITAL DETAILS

Hospital Name

Address

Phone Number

Visiting Hours

Overnight Plan

Notes

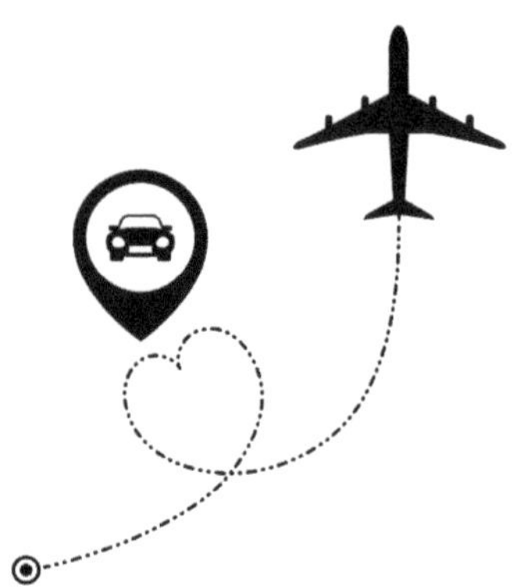

TIME TO GET ON THE ROAD!

We're headed to:

Because:

SURROGACY

Tuck your ticket stub here:

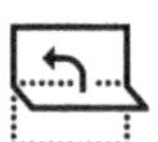

1. ✂   3.   2. ✂

MENTAL HEALTH CHECK IN

Date

Top 3 things we achieved:

Most rewarding thing:

We have felt:

Our three most dominant emotions were:

We are grateful for:

We rate this time period as:

We are working on:

DELIVERY DAY

We're here! Pinch me. Or yourselves.

For you, this day may have been planned for months, or it may have come up very suddenly. You may be looking forward to a smooth birth, or it might be a rocky start. Remember that all emotions are valid.

It's easy to get carried away, but here's some things to think about:

- Support your GC and their wellbeing
- Check what they are comfortable with being filmed and photographed
- Communicate clearly with hospital staff so they know who you are and your roles
- Be prepared for the unexpected
- Document the occasion (we have a whole chapter for this in the coming pages)
- Celebrate!

As you go through this process, note your emotions, tensions and reflect on your relationship with each other and your GC and their loved ones below.

DELIVERY DAY CONT.

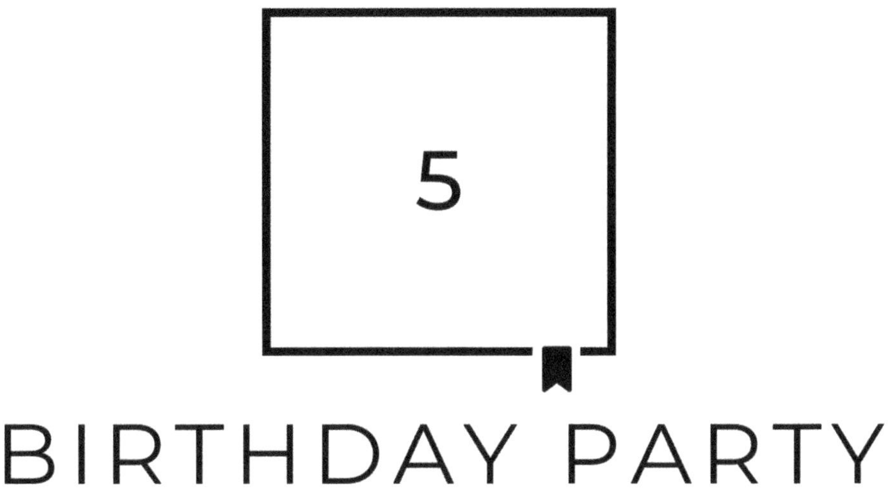

5

BIRTHDAY PARTY

Collect some memories.

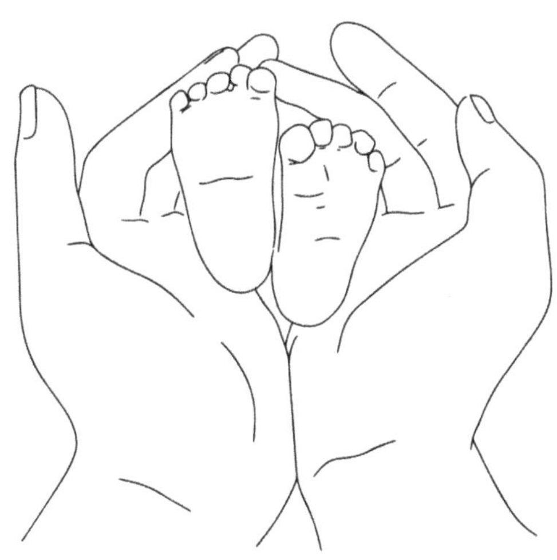

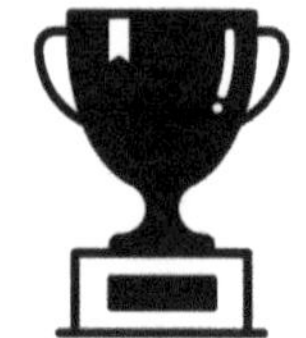

YOU'RE DADS

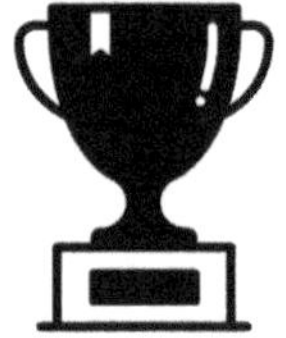

CONGRATULATIONS!

Date

Just bask in it. Seriously.
Big love and hugs.

BABY'S FIRST PICTURE

Date	
Time	
Place	
Time in Labor	
Length	
Weight	

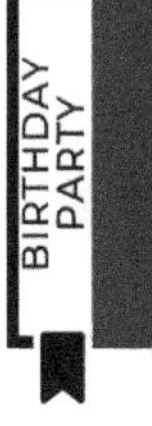

FAMILY PHOTO

Also on this day...

Moments in history

Famous birthdays

BIRTHDAY PARTY

Notable smells

Notable sights

Notable sounds

What was the weather like?

Other things to remember...

BIRTHDAY NEWSPAPER

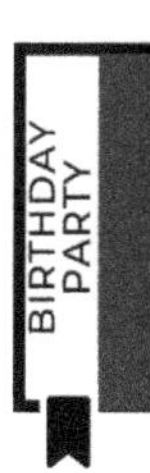

JAN	FEB	MAR	APR	MAY	JUN	JUL	AUG	SEP	OCT	NOV	DEC

1 2 3 4 5 6 7 8 9 10 11 12 13 14 15 16 17 18 19 20 21 22 23 24 25 26 27 28 29 30 31

MENTAL HEALTH CHECK IN

Date ______________________

Top 3 things we achieved:

____

____

____

We have felt:

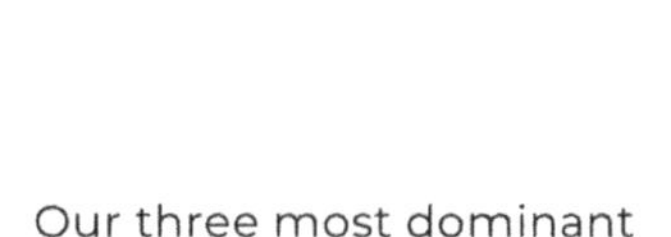

Most rewarding thing:

Our three most dominant emotions were:

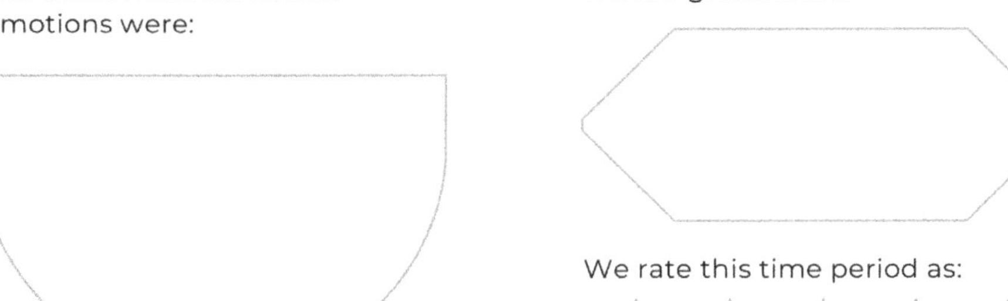

We are grateful for:

We rate this time period as:

⭐ ⭐ ⭐ ⭐ ⭐

We are working on:

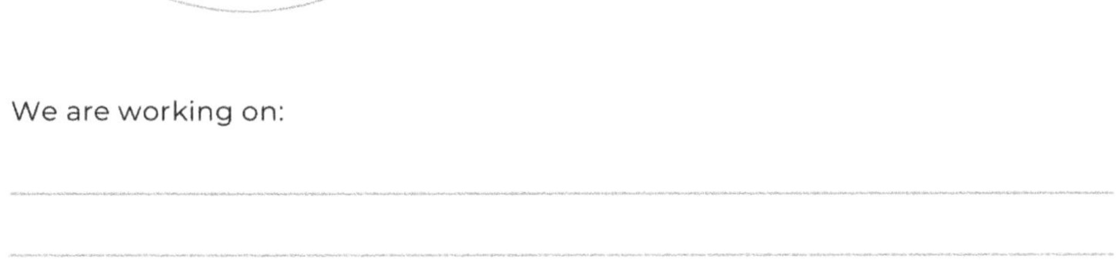

____

____

A LETTER TO YOUR CHILD

You're here. You made it!

This is only the beginning of your overall journey, but to get here was a long trek, in and of itself. I'm sure it was difficult, at times. Once the dust has settled on moving in your new roommate, take some time to reflect by reviewing your entries in this journal.

I hope you both feel proud of your resilience, teamwork and love. Just look at what that love created!

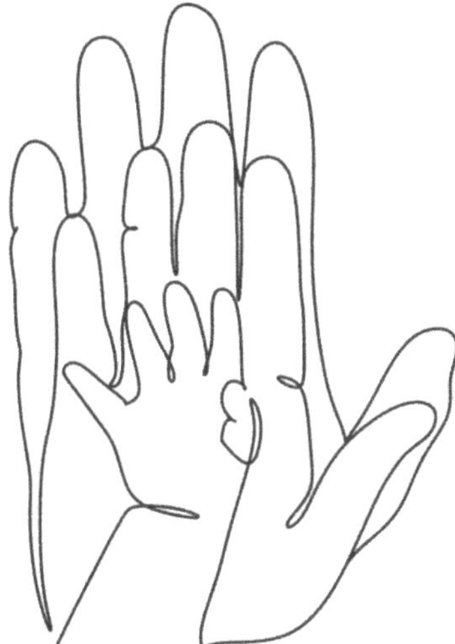

As we wrap up on our time in this journal, I have one favor to ask: consider giving back to your community. After going through something as monumental as you have, wouldn't it be great if you could help just one other person with it? If we could all pass it forward, the world will be an exponentially better place.

That's why I created this journal and I hope it inspires you to give a little, too.

Big love and hugs. And congratulations!

Dave

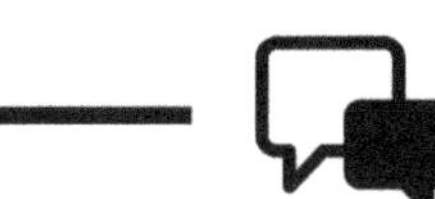

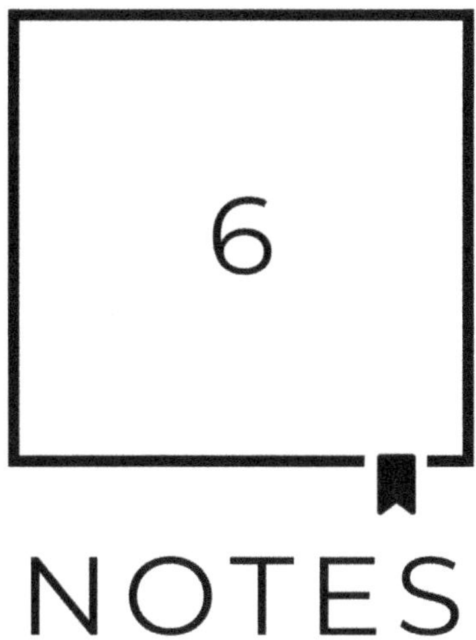

6

NOTES

A space for you to make space.

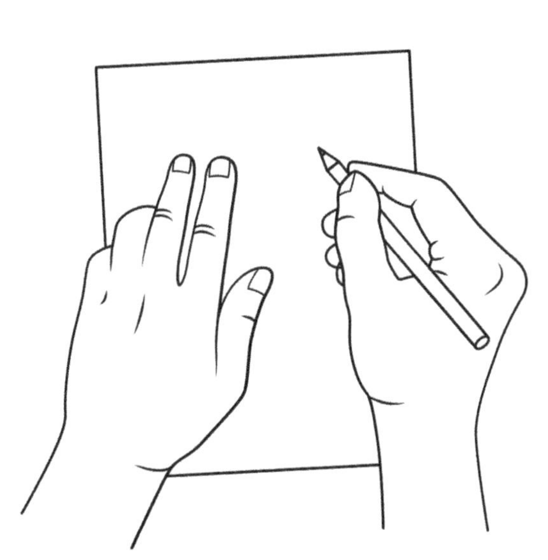

IMPORTANT CONTACTS

Egg Donor

Name

Phone

Email

Address

Gestational Carrier

Name

Phone

Email

Address

Clinic

Name

Phone

Email

Address

Egg Agency

Name

Phone

Email

Address

Surrogacy Agency

Name

Phone

Email

Address

Lawyer

Name

Phone

Email

Address

Psychologist

Name

Phone

Email

Address

Hospital

Name

Phone

Email

Address

IMPORTANT CONTACTS

Name

Phone

Email

Address

Name

Phone

Email

Address

Name

Phone

Email

Address

Name

Phone

Email

Address

Name

Phone

Email

Address

Name

Phone

Email

Address

Name

Phone

Email

Address

Name

Phone

Email

Address

IMPORTANT CONTACTS

Name

Phone

Email

Address

Name

Phone

Email

Address

Name

Phone

Email

Address

Name

Phone

Email

Address

Name

Phone

Email

Address

Name

Phone

Email

Address

Name

Phone

Email

Address

Name

Phone

Email

Address

IMPORTANT CONTACTS

Name
Phone
Email
Address

Name
Phone
Email
Address

Name
Phone
Email
Address

Name
Phone
Email
Address

Name
Phone
Email
Address

Name
Phone
Email
Address

Name
Phone
Email
Address

Name
Phone
Email
Address

NOTES

JAN	FEB	MAR	APR	MAY	JUN	JUL	AUG	SEP	OCT	NOV	DEC

1 2 3 4 5 6 7 8 9 10 11 12 13 14 15 16 17 18 19 20 21 22 23 24 25 26 27 28 29 30 31

JAN	FEB	MAR	APR	MAY	JUN	JUL	AUG	SEP	OCT	NOV	DEC

1 2 3 4 5 6 7 8 9 10 11 12 13 14 15 16 17 18 19 20 21 22 23 24 25 26 27 28 29 30 31

<table>
<tr><td>JAN</td><td>FEB</td><td>MAR</td><td>APR</td><td>MAY</td><td>JUN</td><td>JUL</td><td>AUG</td><td>SEP</td><td>OCT</td><td>NOV</td><td>DEC</td></tr>
</table>

1 2 3 4 5 6 7 8 9 10 11 12 13 14 15 16 17 18 19 20 21 22 23 24 25 26 27 28 29 30 31

<table><tr><td>JAN</td><td>FEB</td><td>MAR</td><td>APR</td><td>MAY</td><td>JUN</td><td>JUL</td><td>AUG</td><td>SEP</td><td>OCT</td><td>NOV</td><td>DEC</td></tr></table>

1 2 3 4 5 6 7 8 9 10 11 12 13 14 15 16 17 18 19 20 21 22 23 24 25 26 27 28 29 30 31

JAN	FEB	MAR	APR	MAY	JUN	JUL	AUG	SEP	OCT	NOV	DEC

1 2 3 4 5 6 7 8 9 10 11 12 13 14 15 16 17 18 19 20 21 22 23 24 25 26 27 28 29 30 31

THANKS

Special thanks to the following for reviewing and editing the drafts of this journal:

- Dawn Baker - CEO, US Surrogacy LLC
- Amira Hasenbush, Esq. - All Family Legal
- Dr. Nurit Winkler, MD - Los Angeles Reproductive Center
- Caitlyn Devine - Intended Parent Case Manager, Center for Surrogate Parenting
- Brian Blitzer - Benefits Coordinator, Men Having Babies
- Don Weiner, Successful Parent through Surrogacy

Thanks also to my beautiful family. To my husband Mathew for navigating this incredible life with me and inspiring me to be a better human, every day. There is nobody that I would want to be sharing these adventures with than you.

To my sister, Rachel, for donating her eggs to our surrogacy journey. I think you understand how important that was to us, but I am not going to stop saying it!

To both Mathew and Rachel for contributing to ideas during long car rides to and from the clinic. You talked sense into me and created ideas that I hadn't even thought of. Thank you!

To my extended family for instilling a sense of right and wrong which helped me realize the need for this journal. Thank you for being my ground.

Finally, thanks in advance to you all for spreading the love and doing something good.

If you have any feedback for future editions or ideas for other publications that are needed, please reach out at publishing@supercreative.global.

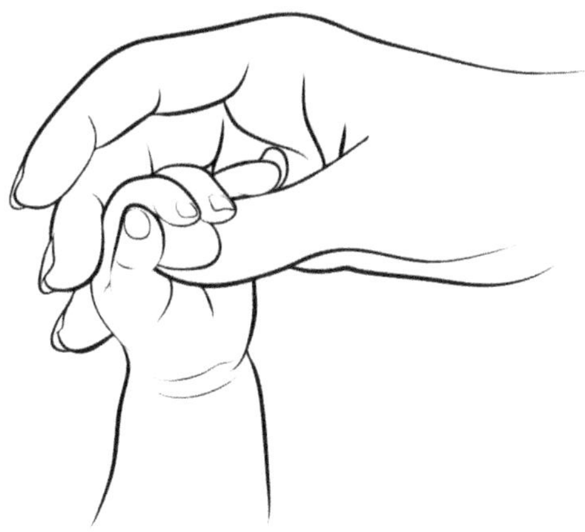

Thank you to all of the artists on Canva who made creating this journal and getting it into your hands so much faster.